I0439402

A Smoker's Revelation

Quit Tobacco and Cut Back on Marijuana

Gerald Shingleton

Copyright © 2014 CadArm Publications

ISBN: 10 1497387655
ISBN-13:978-1497387652

NOTICE:

This document is geared towards providing exact and reliable information in regards to the topic and issue covered. The publication is sold with the idea that the publisher is not required to render accounting, officially permitted, or otherwise, qualified services. If advice is necessary, legal or professional, a practiced individual in the profession should be ordered - From a Declaration of Principles which was accepted and approved equally by a Committee of the American Bar Association and a Committee of Publishers and Associations.

The information provided herein is stated to be truthful and consistent, in that any liability, in terms of inattention or otherwise, by any usage or abuse of any policies, processes, or directions contained within is the solitary and utter responsibility of the recipient reader. Under no circumstances will any legal responsibility or blame be held against the publisher for any reparation, damages, or monetary loss due to the information herein, either directly or indirectly.

The information herein is offered for informational purposes solely, and is universal as so. The presentation of the information is without contract or any type of guarantee assurance.

The trademarks that are used are without any consent, and the publication of the trademark is without permission or backing by the trademark owner. All trademarks and brands within this book are for clarifying purposes only and are the owned by the owners themselves, not affiliated with this document.

TABLE OF CONTENTS

INTRODUCTION

Thank you for choosing this book. Most likely you are a smoker, know it is harmful, and want to quit. I used tobacco products for about twelve years before quitting. It wasn't easy, but I had a method that worked for me and it could work for you as well. Back in the late 60's and early 70's when I evolved into a rather heavy user, pot smoking acquaintances were offended by my foul habit. It never dawned on them that smoke, any type, certainly could have harmful elements. They were right though, tobacco happens to be far worse than Cannabis.

There's a lot of controversy lately concerning high praise for marijuana and just how terrible tobacco is. Stores are even banning cigarette sales. Meanwhile "pot-shops" are opening up all over where states have legalized the drug, both recreationally and medically.

Conservatives do not understand vicious attacks on tobacco while *pot* is highly praised, going back to the Woodstock days. Bill O'Reilly believes there's hypocrisy. An interview with Dennis Miller on the O'Reilly Factor, March 19, 2014, demonstrated this paradox. "Let's just cut to the chase and make pot mandatory." Miller claimed.

Miller said he always rejected tobacco, except maybe when he was a kid just fooling around. The idea of dirty vapors entering his lungs seemed repulsive and disgusting. "I just can't imagine my lungs rotting away from smoke. If you say you need education and claim you don't know tobacco is bad, you're lying through the hole in your trachea. Everybody knows smoking is bad for you."

Bill O'Reilly reminded the listeners that in the 40's and 50's, no one claimed dangers of smoking. "I was a second-hand smoke victim growing up. I was sitting in the back seat of our Nash Rambler with my sister in a thick cloud. It looked like Hiroshima in there."

"Life happens." Miller responded. "If you want to smoke – Smoke! If you do not – Don't." He continued to explain simple facts. "There are three things that can happen when lighting up where *no-smoking* is posted; someone will tell you to put it out, the guy next to you may go to the management and complain, or someone can sucker punch you."

Most don't understand how our government can spend billions on writing a convoluted health care act and then introduce bills to decriminalize or even legitimize marijuana and restrict tobacco use. That's an interesting topic for discussion, yet there's a whole lot of people who stick to their guns defending the Cannabis drug. In fact here's two memos written to the O'Reilly factor on March 19, 2014.

"Cigarettes vs. pot is not a legitimate comparison. Cigarettes have no redeeming qualities while marijuana relaxes people and helps medically." Janet West, Long Beach, CA.

"Casual pot use is relatively harmless. Abusing any substance is dangerous." Dr. Mike Jenkins, North Logan, UT.

Perhaps there's legitimacy in these claims. The cautionary tale of "reefer-madness" is over. The effects of marijuana have been studied to death and facts speak for themselves. But there are issues to explore and it's quite fascinating comparing the two plants, tobacco and Cannabis.

Almost everyone recalls the propaganda explosion and melodramatic events when high school students were lured by marijuana pushers. Interestingly enough, view have dramatically changed. The nation's first medical marijuana advertisement occurred on March 07, 2014, from New Jersey and Illinois with commercial spots scheduled for Massachusetts. The actor professionally portrayed a drug dealer dressed in a heavy trench coat filled with inside pockets and hangers to display products when opened up.

"Yo, you want Sushi? I got Sushi. I got the best Sushi. This area is dry. You know that and I know that. No one knows better than me. I've got tuna and salmon. I got the finest sashimi anywhere. You need me and I need you. Let's make this work. You buy sashimi and I'll throw in some rice paper. I have everything, even California Rolls."

A voice in the background makes a definitive statement, sounding like God's commandment from the universe.

"You wouldn't buy your Sushi from this guy, so why would you buy your marijuana from this guy?"

The point made; tobacco smoking commercials are no longer sanctioned or popular. Marijuana, on the other hand, is the new *healthy* smoke and medical advertisements are now even legal, sanctioned, and encouraged.

1 SMOKE

Does something really dangerous happen to your health when inhaling smoke? Are there poisons consumed? Is there a big difference in types of smoke? Is tobacco smoke worse than marijuana? If you smoke, are you curious what exactly happens to all the workings of your body? Why in the world do millions smoke despite dire warnings?

The argument continues, cigarettes are bad, but marijuana smoke is healthy. That's been the mantra all the way back to the flower children of the sixties. Today, state governments are legalizing the plant because their research finds favor in medical and recreational drug use. After all, contemporary reasoning proclaims that there's nothing unhealthy and medical marijuana has many benefits.

For now, let's try to reason health issues and come up with logical suppositions. Now you may disagree with some facts or why I even bring up something that has nothing to do with personal problems, but it is something to think about. Topics are all public health related concerns.

Back in the 60's and early 70's, there was some devastating environmental alarms. I remember horrific pollution that plagued the inland southern California region. There were smog alerts (mixture of fog and smoke), that mandated that children did not participate in physical school activities and stay indoors. The inversion layer sometimes elevated up to the timber line in the surrounding mountain ranges and actually killed pine trees. At that time, pollution was highly toxic to humans and caused severe sickness and shortened life.

Something had to be done. Fortunately, environmental quality has improved tremendously since those days. But now there are even greater concerns about what is happening to our planet. Whether damage is done by mankind or a natural cycle, it doesn't matter. Legislators are convinced something has to be done.

There's all kinds of talk nowadays about *weather* change due to manmade carbon emissions. Politicians are ranting about dangers to our lives and even the doom of civilization unless something drastic is done to stop the global warming and poisoning.

A universal proclamation claims everyone's life is in danger, and drastic measures are at hand, all because damage to the environment is caused by mankind's foolish behavior. You have nothing to say about this either. You can't buy incandescent light bulbs anymore. Yes, life is tough, but what kind of damage is personally done to our personal health? If smoking is bad, and we all know it is, why not just ban tobacco altogether? But can you imagine a mass withdrawal? Think of the consequences.

So, the comparisons are exaggerated perhaps. But the smoke in smog, comes in several varieties. There are a multiple of types but all contain soot particulates. One variety is vehicular emissions from internal combustion engines along with industrial fumes which combine to form dangerous photochemical particulates.

Firemen also learn that smoke is bad. They take advantage of every available technological protection, yet can't help but consume some amounts. Their symptoms range from coughing and vomiting to nausea. They even experience sleepiness and confusion. Sometimes the smoke gets hot causing burns to the nose, mouth and face. Many times there's singed nostril hairs along with breathing difficulty.

Smoke inhalation injury also includes burned saliva (carbonaceous sputum).

Sure, smoke from brush and forest fires are hot and uncomfortable. Still, safety equipment and respiratory protections filters out most harmful heat and particles. And medical treatment depends on the severity though still advised, usually consisting of humidified oxygen, bronchodilators, suction, endotracheal tubes and even chest physiotherapy. In extreme cases, inhalation therapy utilizes nebulized heparin, a sulfide drug. Acetylcysteine intravenous therapy, when used, continues five to seven days during a supervised hospital stay.

Medical professionals claim carbon monoxide is always presumed to be a complication. That's all because smoke from brush, crops, and wood produces a mixture of particles and chemicals produced by incomplete burning of carbon-containing materials. The approach is to flush out the poisons involving special oxygen compounds.

Firemen's long term affects are chronic. Long term exposure to ambient air containing fine particles has been associated with increases in cardiovascular disease and mortality in populations living in high risk fire areas.

Amazing that all this health concerns are devoted to a job related risk. On the other side of the issue, others seek joy and escape by purposely breathing oxygen deprived smoke, filled with harmful particles. There's an irony here and the next chapters will disclose the truth about smoke, recreational, medical, and otherwise.

2 THE REASON TO SMOKE

There's a reason people smoke cigarettes. Have you ever thought about it? Don't kid yourself, the simple reason is actually two-fold. First, they begin in most cases because of the influence of other people who smoked, usually their parents! Once hooked, he or she then continues – not because of the relaxation and relief it affords, but – because of being psychologically, emotionally, and mentally hooked on the drug.

Ironically, there used to be television and magazine cigarette advertisements and commercials. They cleverly featured youth, vitality, excitement, fun, and all those things attractive to young people in particular. Back in the 50's and 60's, youngsters started the habit early, sometimes eight years old. I remember a news article in college (around 1968) indicating that about ten percent of fifth and sixth graders smoked.

Young boys and girls wanted to be grown up. They wanted to be just like mom and dad. They wanted to feel big and important. Those are facts and the basic underlying reasons children start.

The industry targeted youth because getting hooked amounted to a lot of long term profits. They knew damage would be inflicted but money overruled health concerns. Companies understood addiction very well, and glorifying their products was a way to celebrate conquering the weak minded users.

It all boils down to vanity – a desire to exalt and enlarge the Self – to make oneself more important. This is vanity, a condition that cigarette manufactures studied and manipulated to their benefit.

Smokers would eventually crave the effects of nicotine and tars, becoming a whimpering, cringing, crawling, abject slave of the tobacco god. The cigarette would become a master. The victim then turned into a worshipful, adoring, and trembling servant.

So if you are a smoker, the real reason you began and have continued, is not because you really enjoy them, right? No, be honest with yourself. Sure, you may believe smoking helps relax you, relieves anxiety and tension, but does it? You probably began for much of the same reasons described. Too many are victims of society. You most likely followed the herd like dumb sheep.

Evidence reveals a different outcome. Smoking actually becomes a vicious cycle – it <u>adds</u> to anxiety and increases tension. People who claim that smoking calms their nerves is one big lie. Nervous smokers want to relieve tension but the effects are only temporary.

If one has a need for a cigarette, it is because they became a psychological and chemically addictive slave to a toxicant. This necessity proves that the poisons have started their deadly work. The more a person continues to whip the nervous system, the more nerves become abnormal. All that the tobacco does is appease the craving of the addict.

Once you get started, and usually just getting past that difficult initiation stage of nausea and headaches, several types of psychological pleasures develop. Analysis describes forms of individual expressions. Observe for yourself. Look at the way some hold the cigarette. Then watch the oral pleasure, almost like a toddler sucking a thumb. But every person who is hooked develops categorical cigarette personalities. Some examples follow.

Thinking back when I smoked, a five minute break at work was exactly the length of time for one cigarette. In some contrived way, people began comparing the burning down of a cigarette as a function of time, like an hourglass. To me, it was an excuse to take an unscheduled break. Then there was the break room that seemed to turn into a cloud for fifteen minutes a day. That's when I could observe smoking behaviors.

Many non-smokers complain about employees exiting the work environment to catch a smoke. There are so many legislative restrictions concerning smokers, that designated areas are located quite a long distance away from the work station. That means the five minute break has turned into twenty minutes of lost productivity. This is the type of personality hang-up that is crucially devastating to society.

Added to this mixture of behaviors are multitudes of symbolic gestures. Watch someone blow smoke circles. I've witnessed some spectacular formations. One relaxing moment, as a confirmed smoker will attest, is to sit back and blow rings and then blow another through the first one. That's a sign of being perfectly relaxed.

Mannerisms are amazing and innumerable. Some popular examples are the drooping cigarette profiles. Watching this phenomena when I was a kid caused me to imaging wet lips contained some form of glue. Others could engage unique facial muscles. Their talents were intriguing where the cigarette would mysteriously jump up and down in their mouth while talking.

Aggressive men would hold their *stick* with the thumb and forefinger so the glowing end showed toward the palm of their hand. Dignified women would use a holder for a European flare. FDR had that smart and famous profile with a smoke angled upward and away from his face.

Lighting up is curious too. My father never used a lighter. In the evenings, he'd spent time separating paper matches so that a book of twenty could be used for twice as many cigarettes during the day. I don't know if he thought he was saving money or just looking for something to do. Cheap and expensive lighters came in all types and sizes and engaging a flame always turned into a particular personality ritual.

Smoking rituals also include the *pack-tamp*. I never found the need for this. But the experienced users learned from others about this important preparatory undertaking. Packing, as they like to call it, was accomplished by inverting an unopened cigarette pack, and rapping it a total of three times. Loose tobacco was evidently condensed when striking the hand palm or a table. That's theoretical, but it looked clever enough to be convinced something of significance occurred.

I never did this and I don't have a clue if this is still done, but some users are superstitious. They would remove a cigarette from the pack and invert the damn thing. Then they'd replace it upside down. I guess this was for good luck and that stick became the sanctified last stick to smoke.

Then there's that significant coolness in a personality when a tightly packed cigarette is removed by tapping or what is known as the finger rap, which dislodges the cancer stick so the smoker's lips can reach it. You see, there's a rather unusual implication demonstrated, by celebrating an act where one removes the emerging cigarette with teeth and lips, rather than by nicotine stained fingers.

The cigarette *stick hold*, explains a lot about personalities. It's fun to label people. But seriously, during WWII, this was a key way to uncover spies. The Germans couldn't break the habit. Americans called it the *Euro II*, cigarette hold. But the Germans could uncover American spies too. They could be singled out because of their unbreakable *Classic* stick hold.

Just for fun, you can "google" *cigarette-holds* and find interesting Smoker's Psychology on the internet. There are plenty of old magazine articles that go to extremes explaining gestures, walks, sits, hand motions, and associated nervous habits that develop as a result of being a smoker.

A necessary procedure is the ash flicking. When the burning end of the stick remains on the tip, at some point the fine gray ash needs removal. At that point, the inappropriate act would be to allow it to hit the floor or ground. That's why ash trays were cleverly designed to accommodate the flick. Some have formed a self-made flick with their fingers while others tap the end on the device for proper removal.

During my college days, I fallaciously figured that smoking helped me think. Where deep concentration was necessary, I'd light up. All outside stimuli seemed excluded because of a smoke screen (pun intended).

There are smokers that subconsciously believe that the act has a capacity to *blow troubles away*. I never understood this feeling, but in times of high tension, cigarettes provide relief. It's like an inanimate object becoming a sounding board for your troubles. The cigarette acted like a consolation.

3 SMOKE YOURSELF TO DEATH

My father was one of the fellows who would walk a mile for a Camel. For fifty years, damage slowly deprived him of oxygen. Emphysema goes hard on a man. It was hard watching his last gasp for air.

Extreme cases are evident. I remember one poor father who was in a wheel chair at my high school graduation in 1964 because he lost his right leg due to poor circulation, all caused from smoking.

Doctors back then explained it simply, "Tar and nicotine blocked blood vessels and arteries, just as rust blocks up water pipes, cutting down the flow of blood - causing gangrene."

I believe just about everyone knows someone who died prematurely due to smoking. My cousin died from coronary disease and had a year's supply of nicotine gum in her closets. Her husband passed away from lung cancer, twenty years before. My uncle died from smoking as well. There's universal advice commonly available and repeated here. "If you haven't smoked – don't start. If you do smoke – quit. Don't be a looser."

Whether pleas and this story will stop anyone from smoking, I do not know. I seriously doubt it. Not a single soul I've preached to has quit. Not a single one. Everyone thinks that bad health happens to the other guy, never to them, so they want to believe. But there comes a time when it's too late. It may not be too late for you though! And if you think that marijuana is not a bit harmful, continue reading.

Undesirable side effects of Cannabis includes a decrease in short-term memory, dry mouth, impaired motor skills, reddening of the eyes, and feelings of paranoia or anxiety. Overdosing happens too. I know, because I was summand, from a deep sleep, to take a victim to the emergency room. I remember the incident well, at 3 am in a snow blizzard. Evidently the brownies were so good, she had seconds and thirds and who knows. Unfortunately for me, I too had one or two and was in a state of extreme paranoia. Arriving at the emergency room was truly scary. Sheriffs were there accompanying a rape victim. The problem was, I knew the gal and that made matters worse.

Functional imaging studies have revealed morphological brain alterations in long-term Cannabis users. Reports state some facts about *Resting Blood Flow* - lowering globally in prefrontal brain areas.

The alarms go off when discovering teenagers losing eight IQ points from childhood to adulthood. And the younger they were when they started smoking, the greater the IQ decline. One conclusion stated that marijuana may permanently hurt the developing teen brain.

The peculiar thing about this drug is the fact that after a certain age, marijuana triggers neurogenesis, which means it actually leads to brain cell growth. So there's something unusual about brain chemistry and Cannabis.

Sooner or later, the way I see it happening, the smoke breaks at work will start to include pot (more and more). There will be glares, arguments, and psychological fights between the two different user types. I doubt if fights will ever occur; tobacco users are tough but weak and pot makes you too mellow to engage.

Personally, I look at marijuana like alcohol. Used sparingly, there's probably no health risks or at least minimal. In fact, like a small glass of red wine for dinner, marijuana has positive medical advantages. But anything can be abused. And if you find yourself addicted, maybe it is time to seriously consider quitting. I think that's good advice for any addict, drugs or alcohol.

Tobacco Chemistry:

There are 300 different chemical compounds in tobacco smoke. One puff contains 15 billion particles. Many materials are the most noxious substances known to mankind. A partial list begins with nicotine, pyridine, methyl alcohol, ammonia, carbon monoxide, furfural, and formaldehyde. There are various acids too, like formic, oxalic, citric, acetic, coffeic, and hydrocyanic. You may be surprised to know there's also arsenic, acetone, phenols, and cancerogenic benzopyrene.

Nicotine is one of the quickest, most fatal poisons known. One cigar contains about 100 milligrams. If 500 milligrams of nicotine, according to some medical experts, were directly injected into the bloodstream, the victim would die immediately.

Being carcinogenic, *Tars* have been linked with cancer. This harmful substance is formed during the heating of tobacco. Blow this smoke through a white cotton handkerchief and witness a brown, malodorous stain, evidence of the tars. A smoker who uses about one and one half packs a day deposits a quart of tar annually on the mucous membranes of the mouth, pharynx, larynx and lungs.

One pack a day habit produces and deposits 36 milligrams

of arsenic into the body every year. The arsenic comes from a lead arsenic compound used in some pesticides, an amount legally permitted in food.

Tobacco smoke is deadly. When you smoke, you take *YOUR LIFE* into your own hands, It's a deadly game! Can you really afford to smoke, when you add up all the costs, expenses for cigarettes, medical bills, decreased efficiency, increased nervousness, chronic illness, and ultimately perhaps terminal cancer?

Marijuana (Cannabis sativa) Chemistry:

Plant leaves are psyche-active containing a high concentration of alkaloids – bitter tasting, nitrogen bases. There's also cannabs. One in particular is appropriately identified as cannab- idiotic acid (a fitting name for mind alteration). There are differences around the globe on the percentage of THC (tetrahydrocannabinol) ranging from 1 to 20 percent.

There's additional identifiers like a scientific description of a naturally existing isomer of delta 8 or 9-THC. But the molecules actually vary in complexities producing a large variety. In a pure form, without other substances like insecticides, the smoke produced and inhaled does not represent a significant health risk. So far, there has been no reported cases of lung cancer or emphysema attributed to its use.

Medical professionals claim that a day's breathing in any metropolitan area with poor air quality poses more of a threat than inhaling a day's dose (a portion of a joint).

But, let's not just dismiss this. If a daily dose is 3 to 4 Cannabis cigarettes each day, there's associated evidence of acute and chronic bronchitis, about the same as in excess of 20 tobacco cigarettes. The smoke weakens the immune system and there's evidence of lung infections due to particulates in the smoke. Cells get damaged that line the bronchial passage. Results are impairment of the principal immune cells in the small air sacs.

Now in the case of treating AIDS, patients receiving marijuana pills have improved immune functions. They also gain weight where they could not without the drug. Patients with preexisting immune deficits due to AIDS should be expected to be vulnerable to serious harm caused by smoking marijuana, however. Pros and cons are all over the internet for further investigation.

For one thing, people smoke to get high. It's more efficient to smoke than swallow or eat – at least getting intoxicated immediately. An experienced smoker who inhales deeply and holds it in a long time will retain up to 80 percent of the cannabinoids inhaled.

You can do internet searches and find an amazing amount of information about the medical benefits of cannabis. Before 1937, marijuana was legal, but the "Reefer-Madness" campaign initiated legislation for its prohibition. Just think how many lives would have been saved if Tobacco-Madness caused the prohibition against nicotine.

4 HOW TO QUIT SMOKING

The emphasis here is for tobacco because marijuana has been determined to only be addictive for about 10 percent of users. But, if you are addicted and want to quit, this exercise applies.

All kinds of gadgets, gimmicks, medicines, and even mysterious potions have historically been offered purporting to assist the smoker in quitting. Nothing is guaranteed effective. Remedies do not work. Gadgets, pills, candy, gum, or even hypnosis fails to do the trick.

The new trend is smoking e-cigarettes. This is a nicotine product. Sure, the tars and harmful substances are eliminated, but realize that the vapors contain an addictive drug. The whole idea of quitting is stepping up to the plate, use your will-power, and win the battle. This may, as a last resort, be a useful tool to quit altogether, but certainly not recommended or advised for combat use.

Sadly, the fact that wars slay thousands, but smoking kills millions, should be all the information necessary to convince anyone to stop their dreadful habit. Think about that for a moment. The chances of dying in war are limited to those who are fighting. But smoking slays people in a stealthy way in every walk of life. Death happens in the relative safety of their own homes.

If you smoke, it isn't easy to just say, "I quit!" The real question that a smoker needs to ask, "Do I really want to enjoy life, its riches, thrills, and delights? Do I want to smell tantalizing aromas, the fragrance of fresh crisp air and the spicy scents of nature?"

Give your lungs a chance. Do you realize that when you stop inhaling foul poisonous particulates, your lungs begin to repair themselves? The damage is reversed. Body defenses come into play. Your internal mechanisms destroy pre-cancerous cells! Lungs slowly and gradually turn pink again. But keep this in mind, one or two cigarettes a day prevents the healing and so does switching to pipes or cigars.

I know what I'm talking about because back in the late 70's, I switched from cigarettes to cigars. You're not supposed to inhale, but I eventually did. Then pipe smoking was tried. I inhaled that as well and got real sick and tired of cleaning the foul dregs from the apparatus. So back to cigarettes and this time more than ever.

My life reminded me of what James the First, King of England, proclaimed in 1604, in his famous Counterblast to Tobacco. "Smoking is a loathsome custom to the eye, hateful to the nose, harmful to the brain, dangerous to the lungs, and in the black stinking fume thereof, nearest resembling of the horrible *Stigian* smoke of the pit that is bottomless." That declaration was made absolutely true – a very serious public health menace!

There are plenty of publications and internet sites regarding Smoking and Health. Public Health Services indicate that millions give up the smoking habit every year. The American Cancer Society publishes impressive annual figures of ex-cigarette smokers in the tens of millions. Figures are very encouraging. If you are not an ex-smoker, do you want to become one? Obviously you can quit. It can be done, but how?

To give you an idea about the range of behavior and

addiction, there's one story that's worth mention. It is remarkable, and she claims it a miracle. This is how my wife quit smoking.

I remember well. She quit when pregnant but after the baby was born, she took up the nasty filthy habit again. She tried keeping it a secret, sneaking around. But with time, the habit got worse, so bad, she was up to three packs a day.

She couldn't keep the secret. After openly admitting her syndrome, she was free to smoke anywhere and anytime. Eventually, something strange and mysterious happened.

On one light-up occasion, she suddenly claimed something was terribly wrong. She said it felt like smoke was inside her brains and causing a horrific pressure. But it went away. That same week, she lit up again and this time the extreme pressure was way too much. She put the cigarette out and shouted, "I quit! That's the last cigarette I'll ever smoke."

Of course I didn't believe it. But after that moment, not a single cigarette ever again touched her lips. In fact, every whiff of tobacco smoke would make her sick. She couldn't believe it herself, no withdrawals, no addiction, no desire to try again whatsoever.

So what are you going to do to quit? What actions are you willing to do? Your very life is in jeopardy. If you have made up your mind that you'll do whatever it takes to quit, read on.

First and foremost to admit, is that slaves to cigarettes, come up with many foolish excuses why they continue to smoke. I've heard them all.

"My time's coming. I'll enjoy smoking until I need to quit."

"No, I'm not going to give it up. I may die young, but I'll be happy."

In my own father's case, he admitted to me, "I can't quit. I just can't."

Here's how to stop, and this is based on my own methods. It's a game, one that you need to win. This works for out of control compulsive smokers! Admit that you are an addict. Scientific reports investigate brain waves of heavy users. Tobacco deprivation causes a drop in frequency of slow brain waves. Abstinence leads to an increase in fast waves of electrical activity which explains why smokers who forgo tobacco feel restless and unable to concentrate.

PHASE ONE:

So step number one is to read all you can about **addiction** and prepare yourself for withdrawal. You'll learn that during the period of abstinence, the pulse slows and blood pressure rises. It is recommended that you consult with a physician, check your vitals, and monitor your health when this particular phase begins. Keep in mind that this is not merely a hard-to-break habit. Most professionals agree that deprivation turns into a significant emotional disturbance.

You will also learn that botanically speaking, you are hooked on a drug, a narcotic. Unlike alcohol or opium, soothing qualities don't take effect until addiction. The soothing qualities is in large measure a relief from the irritation caused by drug cravings. When my wife quit when she became pregnant, she warned everyone on her bowling team to realize her mental state could cause emotional outbursts and crying.

Be prepared! Understand what will be in store. Read as much as you can about symptoms others had gone through when they quit smoking. Realize everyone's body chemistry is different. There could be problems concentrating, headaches, anxiety, and depression.

PHASE TWO:

This step requires admitting that you, as a smoker, rarely face up to realities honestly. Nicotine and marijuana are drugs, plain and simple. As one continues using on a daily bases, you just get used to it. The fact is, the habit just becomes part and parcel to life. The more consumed, the higher and higher the tolerance threshold becomes. The amount of drugs a heavy user can handle amounts to a deadly poison for a non-user.

Marijuana and tobacco are not physically addicting. In other words, stopping will not dangerously effect body performance like heroin or the barbiturates. Nevertheless, it is certainly addicting in the sense of the user becoming dependent, craving its effects, and becoming habituated to its use. Smoking becomes compulsive because of a psychological dependence.

Smokers therefore are not paralyzed devotees. In the back of their minds, they all feel they can quit someday. But human reasoning is very powerful. Some convince themselves they are better off, in an emotional way, to rely heavily on their habit. Basically, a smoker's mind created a bonding, a type of love affair.

It isn't just nicotine. Sure there's a craving, but think of all the developed compulsive behaviors that go along with the habit - the feel of the stick, the sucking, inhaling, the flicking, the break-time events, etc.

Admit it! Smoking satisfies an urgent psychological need. If you smoke (marijuana or tobacco), you believe that the inhaled cloud brings magic to the soul, keeps you calm under tension, and helps cope with a stress-filled life. Convincing yourself of this, makes it even more difficult to abandon the habit.

Once you realize why you smoke, then think of all the reasons why you should not smoke. This begins the third phase of quitting. If you really try, and I suggest writing them all down, you will come up with dozens of great reasons why you should get rid of this disgusting habit.

PHASE THREE:

To get you started, here's a few good reasons to quit. First, there's the threat of lung cancer or other fatal diseases. Second, a nonsmoker has more energy and vitality to enjoy life. Third, the mind functions better. Fourth, and nowadays this is really important, you save a lot of money.

Quitting is a lot more difficult when there's no support. It's hard to do this acting alone. Resources to help you will be friends, family members, and co-workers. Explain how all the associated habits created around nicotine use could even be harder to combat than the addiction.

But here's the biggest of all reasons, prove you have **will-power**. When my father told me he can't quit, I was gravely disappointed. I felt maybe I too inherited his lack of will-power. You want to set a positive example for children and others.

I was able to quit smoking because I looked at a "coffin-nail" and came to an immediate realization that a very small and insignificant physical object gained control of my life. How can a poison dictate my actions? I wasn't about to be conquered by such a small enemy. I knew there was strength within to defeat it.

So this very important step is to conquer the enemy. The war theatre can be well defined. It is after all a serious game. Convince yourself that there's no substitute for victory. Take each and every day as a battlefield. When you face the enemy at the beginning of the day, ask yourself if you are willing to be defeated by the enemy. Are you going to raise the white flag?

If this is where you stop and feel there's no hope, investigate the availability of a *Smoking Cessation Program* in your area. This is a kind of last ditch effort, in my mind. But perhaps a support group will work for you. These programs vary and are usually offered by work place environments, hospitals, health departments, community centers, and religious organizations.

If you really believe this can't even work for you, then there's still hope. I'd research medical associations with expert physicians who can prescribe medications to help you quit. Nicotine replacement therapy also helps and involves a slow reduction in nicotine. Hopefully the cravings decrease with therapy. But I still believe quitting – cold turkey is the best way.

My method was setting daily goals. If only one battle defeat per day would be allowed, decide when exactly that would be? After dinner perhaps? Anxiously counting the minutes in the day are tough, waiting for defeat. But when the battle happens, are you really willing to loose, especially to a small white *gasper*?

There's hope. Remember, smoking is actually a crutch. It

helps users escape tension but with a **fatal** kick-back. In a few days of exhausting battle fatigue, all of a sudden, food tastes better. Your throat stops being clogged with phlegm. You'll get rid of the hacking cough. In about a week, you will feel more nervous, but that tapers off and, surprisingly, you'll even be calmer and more poised.

The battle field gets a little smaller each day. After two weeks, defeating the enemy is at hand. You gain control, but remember, there will be some battles every once in a while and if you do not squash the enemy, you could end up losing, and that may be your life!

Remember, smoking can be defeated. You will begin to enjoy life. Breathing fresh air will be pleasurable. Smelling wonderful aromas of nature will tantalize your olfactory nerves. You'll sleep better. There'll be no more danger of accidents or fires in bed. Smelly butts and roaches will be gone from the house.

All these things will become yours, after you conquer the enemy. Blessings will come and some will be immediately apparent. Think of the benefits of not smoking. Think of the gruesome costs. Sing a victory march in your mind while taking a most enjoyable walk. The lyrics are simple, but effective, "Strong desires, motivation, and resolve to defeat the enemy." Do these things and you will have made a good beginning in stopping. But there's more.

PHASE FIVE:

The final step is to completely overcome the vile, noxious habit. You must plan out your strategy and avoid temptation. You are involved in a major project. Depending on your own psychological makeup, defeat may involve extreme measures of firmness, determination, and tremendous personal effort!

Face up to the fact that quitting triggers more nervousness, tension, and cravings. Face the fact that smoking has a deathlike hold on you. To overcome, it takes time and strategy. There will be suffering, just like any battlefield. But set your goal to win. It can be done.

Always keep goals in mind. Never let it grow hazy, or disappear from view. Don't foolishly put yourself inside a battlefield that can be avoided. You may be tempted to compromise goals. Friends or relatives might persuade you to give in, just once. Chances are, if you do give in, you will be defeated and hooked once again, maybe even worse.

The basic key to defeat the enemy is simple. When you quit, quit completely. Stop all smoking. Use the cold turkey method. Tapering off never works! This failed method only spreads agony over a long period. Tapering down is about as humane as cutting a dog's tail off, an inch at a time, so it won't hurt as much.

Conclusion

I hope this discussion and advice helps you lick this horrible addiction. I know it is hard. My mother-in-law just couldn't stop. She smoked like a chimney. Her environment was filled with nicotine stains. I watched her dwindle and after being diagnosed with cancer, she tried taking the easy way - saving her morphine pills and then consuming enough to end it all.

That didn't work. She ended up almost like a miserable vegetable in hospice. Slowly, she dwindled and passed away. I wished I could have done something, but it was too late. For everyone I've known, and there have been a lot, the slow poisoning from smoking is a horrible thing to witness. I know you can lick it, but you have to make a commitment, recognize the evil, and win on the battlefield. Think about it. That's the **only** way it works.

If you like this read and find it very helpful, please post comments on the Amazon Review for this book. That way, others will be encouraged to read and apply these principles.

Heaven, Can We get There?
Adam and Eve Cosmic Code
Rainbow Caper
Home Baking Business
Home Baking for Profit
Real Estate Math
June Bug
God Power
Finger Pirates
Love Affair in Occupied Japan
Architects Reference Manual
Journey to Terra Incognita
Child Discipline Vs. Spanking